I0469757

It's Hard to Keep Up!

A collection of essays on current topics in
nursing and healthcare from The Blog at
www.nurs-ed.com

By

Cheryl A. Lehman PhD RN CNS-BC RN-BC CRRN

Dedication

To all the nurses before and since.

Preface

This short book of clinically-focused essays, most from **The Blog at www.nurs-ed.com**, may seem like a flight of ideas to some. Perhaps it is – a flight of ideas from an aging mind that is amazed and even confused by the speed at which knowledge in healthcare changes.

I say aging – perhaps a better word is middle-aged – but the mind is in the body of someone – me – who has been a nurse since graduating (the first time) in 1978. And has that mind seen Science explode with new knowledge that affects nursing, healthcare and patient outcomes!

Just think about the last 10 years – the new anticoagulants. The increasing frequency of transplants. C-pap machines everywhere, even on sailboats! Drug-resistant infections. The Affordable Care Act. Increasing patient acuity at all levels of care. The DNP. NPs being accepted as necessary in medical and independent practices coast to coast.

This short ~ 55 page text provides brief updates on nursing and healthcare for practicing nurses who just do not have time to track changes day in and day out. Obesity. Cancer and shiftwork. The microbiome. And many more topics are included in this short book. Most of these do appear as blog entries on nurs-ed.com. So you COULD check them out for free. But there is also material included that has not been published before. Short stories, easily and quickly read, in no particular order, to catch us all up on what the hot topics in healthcare are today.

Our nursing world is changing as we speak. I guess you could say that we are nursing in the "new now". We need to keep up. Thank you for purchasing this book –

thank you for visiting nurs-ed.com. Thank you for being a nurse who wants to keep up.

TABLE OF CONTENTS

Table of Contents

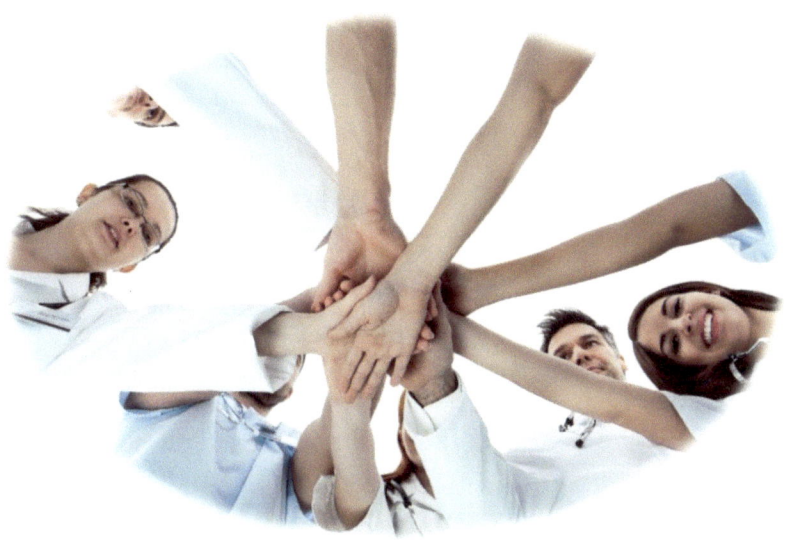

Teamwork

Short stop. Quarterback. Goalie. Center. Which one are you? As the focus on quality grows stronger, healthcare systems are increasingly focused on teams and teamwork. But we didn't start out that way.

Some of us remember when physicians ruled the earth, sort of like dinosaurs. And just like T-Rex, they were bigger, stronger and had way more political power than nurses. Physicians could get nurses fired, disciplined or reassigned. Administrators kissed their feet. Nurses, of course, walked two steps behind, carried the charts for the doctor, gave up their seat for him when he entered, and got him coffee if he needed it. Those were the days. We should cherish them......

Or not, eh? The playing field is now more even. And better for the patient.

There is a growing amount of evidence that when interprofessional teams are functioning well, patients experience less morbidity and mortality. Less illness and fewer deaths when more heads are involved in care. Wow. And also those things that admin loves - shorter length of stay and fewer patient complaints.

Think about it. If an interprofessional team is caring for you, you as the patient will have better outcomes. But, you say, we can't do that! No time. Just give us some orders and we will carry them out. End of story.

It is funny how many nursing students enter college thinking that they will do what the doctor says, no more, no less, no thought. That the doctors are like those on Gray's Anatomy, having sex like rabbits in closets and on-call rooms, and throwing out the occasional order to the nurses. IV STAT! CALL A CODE! GET HIM TO THE OR! NOW!!! And that they, as nurses, will not think or contribute, but will wear their cute scrubs and do what the doctor says. Just like in the old days.

But patient care is now all about interprofessional teams. I have seen teams in action in acute care, rehabilitation and ICU. And they work. In our acute care gero unit, we had sit-down rounds Monday - Friday, with nurses, doctors, social workers, pharmacist, dietitian, PT and OT present. All patients were discussed - on our unit, we had 2 meetings daily - one for the East hall (20 patients), one for the West (30 patients). Meetings lasted 1 hour. Team members came and went as needed. Reports were succinct and to the point - no gossip. And we shared - information on illness, medical plans, medications, function, nursing and social and psych aspects, and discharge planning. And then we briskly moved on to the next patient - and everyone was on the same page and knew the plan without having to read the chart or track someone down.

Our surgical-trauma ICU at that hospital also had team rounds daily - in the morning - intensivist, nurses, therapists (PT, Respiratory), chaplain - and, again, to get everyone on the same page with the plans and progress.

And rehabilitation is one of the settings where team function is traditional, long-standing and pretty much dictated by accrediting agencies, with rounds at least weekly that include the patient and family. Rehabilitation settings somewhat smugly KNOW that teams are valuable!

Team effect on patient outcomes is pretty much a function of synergy. $1+1 = 3$. Think of all of the vast, broad knowledge and experience a single team has...and if the members are open to suggestions and constructive criticism and working together for the good of the patient, magic happens. One team, in and of itself, will have the collective knowledge of PT, OT, MD, RN, SW, Dietitian, PharmD - and all of their combined years of experience. You can see how that collective knowledge and experience makes $1+1 = 3$.

Here are 2 possible scenarios illustrating the value of "team"- both of which are quite common in the US today.

1. Dr. Jones has completed a hip replacement on Ms. Foster, an 89 year old lady. She has been getting PT in the main gym, and is doing well, walking 50 feet with the walker. He tells the team to discharge her tomorrow to home. The social worker visits Ms. Foster and learns that she lives alone, in a house with 12 steps at entry, and then another 10 steps inside to get to the bedroom and only bathroom. Discharge is delayed one week as arrangements are made for SNF care, as SNF beds are limited in Ms. Foster's area. During that week, Ms. Foster develops a UTI

and delirium, and requires antibiotic treatment and antianxiety meds. Her total LOS is 10 days.

2. Dr. Smith evaluates Ms. Foster for a hip replacement, and plans it for next week. In his office, before surgery, she is interviewed by the Nurse Practitioner, who learns that Ms. Foster has 12 steps at entry to her home, and that her bathroom and bedrooms are on the second floor. She has been barely managing her environment up to now, because of her hip pain and limited range of motion. She also notes that Ms. Foster is socially isolated, without access to a car or transportation postoperatively. The NP discusses the case with the PT, who evaluates Ms. Foster and estimates that she will need 4-6 weeks postop to become independent and drive again. The NP also calls the PCP, who tells her a bit more about Ms. Foster's medical and social background, and who suggests SNF care postoperatively. The NP has the social worker see Ms. Foster, explore her funding options, and help pre-arrange for SNF care. The MD, NP, SW and PT meet briefly to discuss the case. Ms. Foster has her surgery as planned, and her LOS in the hospital is 3 days. She is discharged to SNF. She has no complications.

Moral of the story - teams work and make the patient's outcome better.

We as nurses have a responsibility to the function of our particular team - being available, sharing our insight and suggestions, knowing the team plan, contributing to team effectiveness - and being an equal partner in the team. We need to have skills that help us communicate - share - collaborate. And if our environments do not currently have, or support, "teams" - we need to intervene. Get formal interprofessional patient care teams, with regular meetings and functions, implemented in your setting. It's "evidence-based practice"!

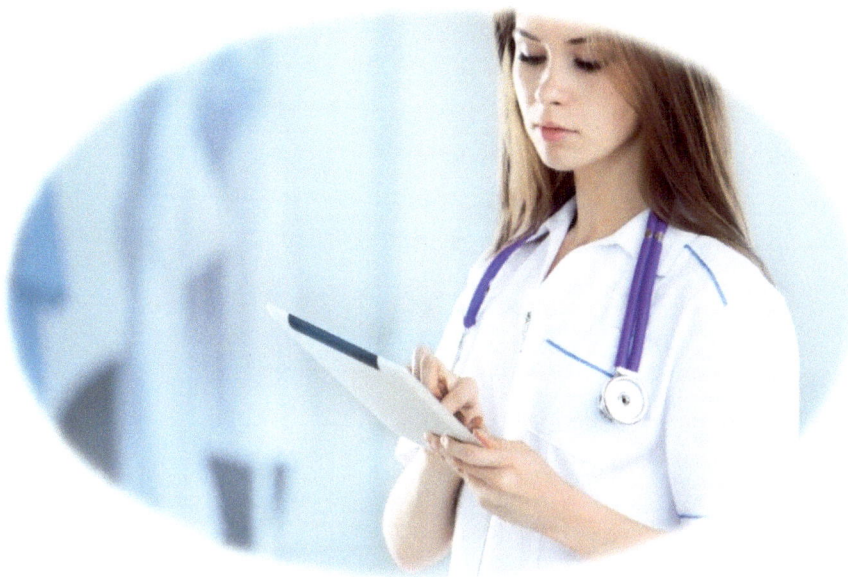

10 ways to cope with being a nurse

AWWWWWK! You have just decided that you hate nursing. You are either:

1. A nursing student who has already invested beaucoup $$ in your nursing education

2. A new nurse with culture shock

3. An experienced nurse who is burnt out

What do you do?

Here are 10 suggestions to keep you in nursing, and keep you happy.

1. *Find a mentor*. Look for a nurse who seems to be happy in their job. Explain your issues to them, and ask for

their help in sorting out your feelings and in making plans for the future. Ask them what they like about their job. What makes them enthused to come to work every day? Did they ever have a time when they considered leaving nursing and finding another profession? How did they handle that? Are they always happy at work, and if not, how do they cope on the bad days? Work with your mentor over time to identify YOUR happy times. Surely there have been one or two! And then work to make those times come again, with your mentor's guidance.

2. ***Examine your work/school/life closely***. Are they separate or overlapping? Do you ever get a break, time just for you? Do you have hobbies, non-nurse friends? Have you drifted away from your faith practices and need to drift back? Work at separating "nurse" from "you", so that you get some down time in a way that allows refreshing and renewing. Vacations. Massages. Pedicures. Piano lessons. An occasional karaoke night! A good meal (yup, don't forget to eat!). Time at the gym. Take your days off. Take your vacations. You have earned them! Don't forget that you can have a life outside of nursing or school. Too many people are work-sleep-work-sleep. We all need a break!

3. ***Think about invoking change***. Nursing students, you are probably out of luck on this one, but practicing nurses: think about a different shift, a different unit, a different specialty. Change can refresh your excitement with nursing. You might want to think about advancing at work, from staff nurse to educator, case manager,

administration. Or, do a lateral move to another unit. One of my early moves was from a med-surg unit where I was assigned 30 patients per night to an intermediate care unit where I was assigned 4. The acuity was higher, but the patient load was less to accommodate it. And I had the opportunity to learn and add depth to my nursing knowledge!

4. ***Expand your network*** - join a professional nursing organization. There are professional nursing organizations such as Sigma Theta Tau International, which is nursing's honor society. STTI is most often joined when you are a student, but can be joined as a "community member" after graduation, as well. There are clinical specialty organizations - for instance, ARN for rehabilitation nurses, AMSN for med-surg nurses, AACN for critical care nurses....just look around on Google for organizations related to your specialty, be it pedi, OB, ortho, plastics, vascular, oncology, whatever. And then join, and volunteer to become involved in org. activities. The national/international networking can be exciting. And I have heard hundreds of nurses, over the years, exclaim how renewed they feel after attending the annual organization's conference! I personally have gained so many leadership skills, so many friends, so many advisors, and so much knowledge from my involvement in STTI, ARN and AANN.

5. ***Consider a return to school*** (sorry again, students!). A wise friend once told me to be smart and

realize that I already had 10 years invested in nursing - why would I consider leaving it (and he was an engineer!). He was right. So I went back to school, and went back to school, and went back to school a 3rd time, ending up with a BSN, an MSN, and a PhD. And a vision, and goals, and renewed excitement in being a nurse. And, although I had thought I already knew everything there was to know, well.....I had a whole lot to learn! And school was fun! Higher education is important for nurses, as is lifelong learning. My newest educational effort is an online Medical Spanish course, worth something like 54 CNE - it will take a while to complete, but the knowledge will serve me well as I embark on a new phase of life - I am soon to begin volunteering as an RN for a local free clinic. And, if you are not interested in higher nursing education, there as associated programs such as Medical Humanities, and others. And.....the online universities and MOOCS - I like Coursera and edx.

6. *Students - this one's for you*. You already have hours and hours and $$ invested. And, if your grades are good, and you still do not think that you will like being a nurse, remember this - there are dozens and dozens of specialties in nursing. These can be clinical specialties - so, you didn't like, pedi, well, work with adults! You didn't like dealing with IVs? Aim toward a clinic practice. You hated dealing with adult diapers? Work in IT with EMR development. Take the time to investigate the possibilities. Stick it out in school. And then work to gain knowledge in the specialty that you want - which may require more

education. I am going to say this - a couple of years in clinical practice will be a great foundation for any specialty that you select within nursing, if you can handle it. It will give you a baseline of knowledge, and a level of credibility that is very useful to have.

7. *Volunteer to become involved at work*. Nursing councils, QI projects, policy development, even managing the unit parties. Precepting student nurses for the semester is another fun assignment. Developing educational activities for your peers. There are many activities that need nurses to become involved. Becoming involved makes you more invested in your workplace. And being more invested in your workplace, and with your peers, gives you time away from your usual duties, giving you a break. It is refreshing and invigorating. Talk to your manager, and see if there is a project that you can become involved in.

8. **Ignore the naysayers and the negative Nellies at work or school.** Negativity breeds discontent and major heartburn. If your BFF at work or in school is the most negative person on the planet, you need a change. Far, far away. Change Shifts! Change Units! Change Seats! Yeah, perky people can be annoying, but have you noticed that they are happy? Happiness can rub off too, making work and school oh so more tolerable. Send Nelly into the stratosphere, and save yourself!

9. *Join a support group. Or start one*! You are not the only one who sometimes feels hopeless, and not the only one who wants to become a fisherman instead of a

nurse. Groups exist on the web, but you may be more comfortable with a local one. Students, you can seek personal counseling at school. Remember that groups should have a purpose, and need to be more than griping and complaining - which is why a professional group leader may be of benefit. Talk to your manager, the hospital chaplain, the social worker, or your nursing faculty about developing a support system for nurses who feel like you.

10. ***Don't worry!*** Sometimes we become dissatisfied with nursing because we feel out of our depth, like we are drowning. Maybe we don't know enough, and might hurt a patient! Maybe we gave the wrong med, and stay up all night worrying about it! Maybe we feel like an idiot when we hear the interprofessional team discussing a patient, unsure of what all of their specialty jargon means. Maybe we slept through patho and pharm and the lack of knowledge is catching up. Maybe we are an imposter!

Most everyone goes through this stage. And there are a few things you can do to decrease your worry and sleepless nights. First, identify the source of your worry, then address it directly. Is it knowledge? Self-confidence? Peers and co-workers?

If you feel you are lacking in knowledge, go and find it! Google. Professional websites. The library. Journals. Admit when you do not know something, and then fix your lack of knowledge! "Sally, I am sorry, but I do not understand the phrase detrusor dyssynergia. Could you explain it to me?" It will be worse if you fake it, and a patient gets hurt. Admitting ignorance trumps bravado every time. And my personal observation is that the more educated the person, the more they will freely admit "I don't know" and seek to remedy the situation. They don't stay up all night worrying, because they stopped, got the needed information, and continued on. And I have heard experienced physicians compliment healthcare workers who ask for explanation or clarification of an order or a concept, because they know how hard it is to admit ignorance, and they admire bravery.

If the problem is self-confidence, talk with your manager about ways to increase your confidence and satisfaction with your work. Regular assessments from the manager and charge nurse can be helpful. And you need to be involved, too, asking for feedback and accepting praise. Self-confidence improves over time, as knowledge, experience and comfort increase.

If the issue is peers and co-workers, again, talk to your manager. The manager is familiar with the staff, and can help you become accepted. We all need to have our co-worker's support, to feel like someone has our back in times of stress and trouble. And we need to support our co-workers as well. It is not always easy to fit into a new group, and it's OK to ask for guidance in how to do so.

If you are feeling the effects of stress, such as sleepless nights, indigestion and heartburn, chest pain, and depression, DO NOT suffer alone. You need to stop! and talk to your mentor and manager immediately. Nursing is not meant to be stressful, or to cause sleeplessness and tears. This is where a support group can help, too. Do not let your job affect your health. And, most important, please do not drown your sorrows with substances to make you forget them - alcohol, prescription and non-prescription drugs. Address the issue at the source - and do not suffer in alone and in silence. Remember, not every nurse can function in every setting. It is OK to admit a problem, and even better to seek help to solve it in a healthful manner.

So, there are 10 suggestions to try to keep you in nursing. We need you! Patients need you! Healthcare needs you! You have a great deal to offer, and you are a valuable member of the healthcare team. If you have an overwhelming need to become a fisherman, do it, but if you are the least bit wishy washy about your decision to leave nursing, give it another chance. I am confident that you can find your niche and be happy. Feel free to call or email me if you would like to discuss this topic in more depth.

Take care!

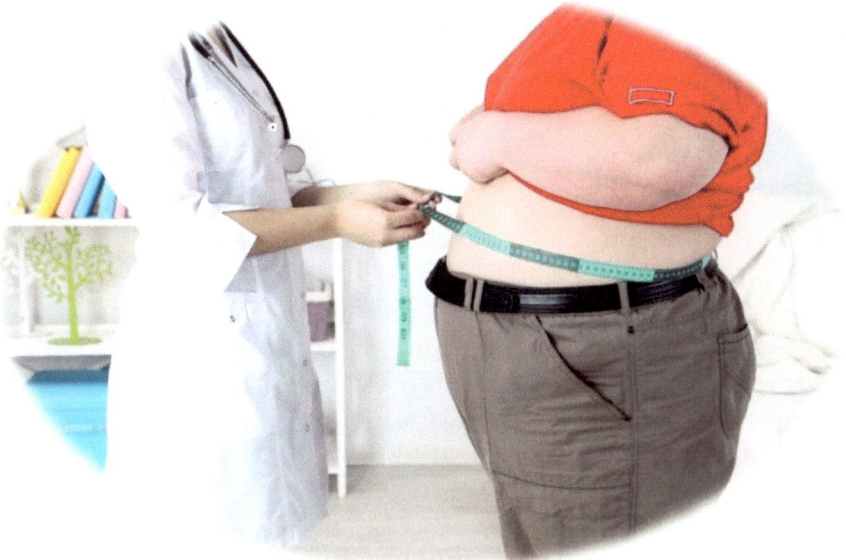

Fat as an active body part

Yup, we're all gaining weight. As an international society. Doesn't matter who or what is to blame - and the thoughts on that are many - fast food. Computer games. Lack of outdoor exercise. Chemicals. Drugs. Pollutants. Hormones. Fear of crime. Whatever. What is most concerning about obesity are the implications of excess body fat.

Did you know that adipose tissue is an active substance? It provides a "microenvironment with concomitant systemic endocrine alterations that favor both tumour [cancer] initiation and progression" (Park, Morley, Kim, Clegg & Scherer, 2014). It is known, in other words, that excess adipose tissue is involved in the development and progression of cancers of the breasts, kidneys, esophagus, GI tract, and male and female reproductive systems. And that's not all. Adipose tissue makes things. Enzymes. Hormones. Cytokines. Growth factors.

Proinflammatory mediators. Adipose tissue helps to regulate appetite, energy balance, lipid metabolism, glucose regulation, inflammation, angiogenesis (growth of new blood vessels), hemostasis (clotting) and blood pressure. And here I just thought it was tasty when cooked on the grill!

There are 2 kinds of fat - white and brown. White is the major form in mammals. Brown is important in thermoregulation and lipid oxidation. WAT (white adipose tissue) is mostly found around the viscera and in sub-q tissue. WAT contains adipocytes, leukocytes, macrophages, fibroblasts, adipose progenitor cells, and endothelial cells. Each adipocyte in WAT contains a large fat droplet occupying 90% of the space, with a few small mitochondria. BAT (brown adipose tissue) has smaller cells, with more fat droplets per cell and larger and more numerous mitochondria. BAT is mostly found around the aorta and is also found around the viscera. BAT has a lot of blood vessels and has a high density of noradrenergic nerve fibers. Where BAT is involved in heat and lipid oxidation, WAT is proinflammatory. It is involved in the development of hypertension and atherosclerosis. In the kidney, WAT is also involved in sodium reabsorption, and thus involved in intravascular volume and renal-associated hypertension. This site: http://themedicalbiochemistrypage.org/adipose-tissue.php has a great table of everything that adipose tissue produces and the actions of each protein or chemical.

Excess adipose tissue increases a person's risk of type 2 diabetes and cardiovascular disease. This, and the increased risk of cancer associated with excess fat, may be due to the presence of inflammation - often associated with obesity. At the cellular level and in the microenvironment, metabolic activity in fat includes insulin resistance, hyperglycemia, dyslipidemia and inflammation. Fat produces adipokines, such as the hormone Leptin. Leptin regulates food intake via the nervous system. As obesity increases, so does the production of Leptin. It is thought that increased levels of Leptin, a hormone that decreases appetite and induces weight LOSS, is involved in dysfunction of Leptin receptors throughout the body, perhaps making them less receptive to binding with Leptin. Thus, Leptin is produced but is ineffective. It is also surmised that increased Leptin levels are associated with the fat-cancer link. Leptin has other activities also affected through the activity of adipose tissue, including regulation of the neuroendocrine axis, bone mass, inflammation, and blood pressure. There is a direct correlation between the high levels of Leptin in an obese individual and the development of atherosclerosis.

Adiponectin is another hormone affected by adipose tissue, but as weight goes up, adiponectin levels go down. Adiponectin is involved in insulin sensitivity and fatty acid oxidation. It is also involved in hemostasis. So, less of the hormone, less insulin sensitivity, less fatty acid oxidation, and more problems with hemostasis. There are other hormones affected in obesity such as Resistin, which increases with obesity. Resistin plays a role in increasing hepatic glucose production through gluconeogenesis and also increases insulin resistance. Resistin is also proinflammatory.

So what? So here are a few examples of the unique effect of fat on health.

Obese children have been found to exhibit higher rates of nonalcoholic fatty liver disease (NAFLD), the most common cause of chronic liver disease in children. This condition can progress through several stages, all the way to cancer. So - obesity can lead from simple steatosis all the way to liver cirrhosis and liver cancer. In kids. It is thought that fat accumulation in the liver leads to inflammation and cirrhosis. Barshop, Francis, Schwimmer and Levine (2009, http://www.ncbi.nlm.nih.gov/pubmed/20556232) note that "Fat accumulation in the liver is likely to result from insulin resistance and concomitant impairment of fatty acid metabolism within liver, skeletal muscle and adipose tissue". There also may be a genetic predisposition to developing the disease when obesity is present, as not all obese children develop NAFLD. But, NAFLD in kids has been associated with significantly higher fasting glucose, insulin, total cholesterol, LDL-cholesterol, TG and systolic and diastolic blood pressure. The problem? Most kids are asymptomatic in the earlier stages, and if not suspected, the disease will be advanced when first identified. Who wants to learn that they need a liver transplant at age 15?

Fat is known to play a role in inflammation in COPD, and the deaths due to cardiovascular dysfunction in that population. Studies have suggested that excess visceral fat in persons with COPD leads to excess IL-6 which leads to increased morbidity and mortality (van den Borst et al., 2012, http://www.ncbi.nlm.nih.gov/pubmed/22811442). Excess abdominal fat in persons with COPD also leads to a mechanical difficulty with breathing, as the fat impedes lung expansion and makes the work of breathing more fatiguing. Abdominal fat, considered to be an indicator of the hidden fat around organs, has been associated with higher risk of heart disease and cancer. And excess abdominal fat has been associated with osteoporosis in men, as well as sleep apnea (http://www.huffingtonpost.com/2013/07/11/belly-fat-heart-disease-cancer-risk_n_3575481.html).

And just think about all of the other diseases associated with obesity. Knee and hip problems requiring joint replacement (and many orthopedic surgeons will not operate on an obese individual, so the pain will continue until weight is lost and surgery is approved by a doctor). Gall bladder disease and gall stones. Gout. Asthma. Pickwickian syndrome. Polycystic ovary syndrome. Dyslipidemia. MI. Stroke. Infertility. And all thought to be caused by the activity of fat - either the physical presence and weight of the fat or the activity of the fat cells. The pathways from obesity to disease are not all clear, other than strong correlations between the presence of obesity and the prevalence of certain diseases. Both the bench research and the clinical research are in full swing, and, as I have said before....we as nurses need to keep an eye on the findings of these studies.

It is likely that in your career you will encounter changes in the medical treatment of persons with obesity that deal with

1. Obesity prevention

2. Weight loss techniques

3. Disease management specific to the presence of excess adipose tissue.

There may be societal changes in diet -- reducing fast foods, improving the cost of foods, fewer hormones in foods and more healthy food supplies with fewer chemicals involved. There may be recommendations in changing our exposures to other chemicals found in our environment - in our furnishings, clothing, meal preparation equipment, medications, air, water. There may be new medications or treatments developed to counteract some of the metabolic activity of adipose tissue. Interventions may be found that work differently in the obese vs the normal weight person. The possibilities are endless.

But first, I think that you will hear of new research findings that dictate the changes in treatment based on what is happening at the cellular level with body fat. And I bet that chronic inflammation associated with obesity will be an important factor, but that other equally important factors will become apparent over time. Stay alert, stay tuned, and keep up to date on the topic. It is sure to affect us all.

Reference:

Park, J., Morley, T. S., Kim, M., Clegg, D.J. & Scherer, P.E. (2014). Obesity and cancer - Mechanisms underlying tumour progression and recurrence. Nat. Rev. Endocrinol. **10,** 455-465.

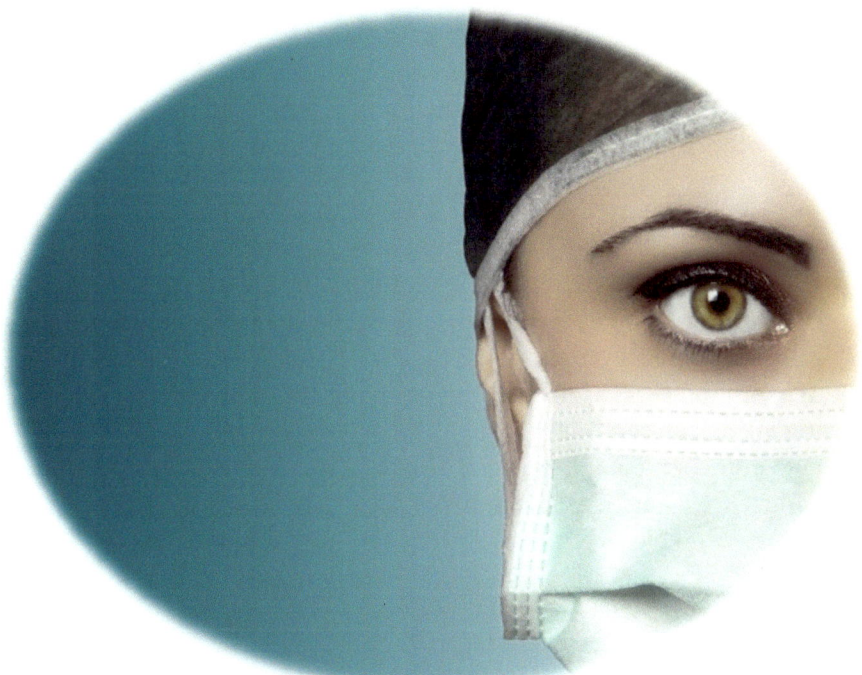

Shift work and health

If you are a nurse, chances are that, sometime in your career, you have worked or will work an "off-shift" schedule - that is, a schedule that includes shifts other than "day shift". In fact, 20-25% of the workforce in industrialized nations is shift workers - in the healthcare, public safety, factory, power supply, and transportation fields, especially.

While, for nurses, off-shift can be a great schedule to work - peace, quiet, patients asleep, managers gone, minimal disruption and chaos - it's not the best for your body. Many nurses are surprised that regularly working an off-shift schedule can affect their health, their life, and even their life-span.

When you work an off-shift, you are probably on a different schedule than your family and friends. Let's face it - most people have normal jobs that are 9-5, 8-4 or even 7-

3. They see the sun. They go to bed after the ten o'clock news. They eat meals at the usual times. They socialize with others who are awake in the daytime.

But when your family is going to bed, you are going to work. And, when you get home in the morning, they are going to work. If you are lucky enough to have the family gone all day, you as the night shift worker can sleep all day - if you can ignore the phone, the computer, the doorbell, the neighbor's lawnmower, the dogs barking at the UPS truck, the cat, the light through the curtains, the guy who comes to fix the air conditioning and the kid who comes home sick from school. What a life! And, on your day off, you try to get back to normal, by sleeping when the family sleeps, and getting up in the morning.

There is an expanding body of research and literature that is beginning to address the health risks of working shift work (anything outside of day shift). Shift work has even been classified as a possible carcinogen by the International Agency for Research on Cancer (IARC), and some countries are compensating workers who developed various cancers while working off shift schedules.

There are 3 basic problems with working off shift - especially the night shift.

1) Sleep and fatigue issues

2) Health problems

3) Traffic and workplace accidents.

I am going to focus on #2 - health issues.

Working the off shift is known to negatively affect the immune, inflammatory and cardiovascular systems.

Workers who work off shifts have also been found to have evidence of epigenetic changes - changes that affect the way that genes work and that can influence disease. Off shift workers have also been found to have more psychological stress, anxiety and depression than day shift workers.

Shift workers have shown evidence of increased cortisol and norepinephrine, increased WBCs, increased C-reactive protein - indicators of stress and inflammation. Shift work is known to increase oxidative stress. Deregulation of circadian rhythms and melatonin disruption is implicated in some of this, but may not be the only cause of health problems.

Shift workers are likely to have lower levels of vitamin D, implicated in development of diabetes. They are also more likely to develop the metabolic syndrome (another diabetes link). It was recently found that shift workers exhibit changes in two substances in the gut - xenin and ghrelin - that control appetite. Shift workers tend to have other dietary issues as well that lead toward obesity.

And if you already have a disease, such as breast cancer? Change in circadian rhythms and melatonin disruption secondary to light exposure at night leads to a known resistance to tamoxifen, a chemo agent used for breast cancer.

So shift workers are more likely to have increased adiposity and obesity, changes in appetite, less vitamin D, more inflammatory markers, impaired sleep, less melatonin, changes in circadian rhythms and a host of yet-unrecognized risk and trigger factors that can lead to diseases such as cardiovascular disease, diabetes, cancer, hypertension, psychological issues....and who knows what all! Teasing out direct cause and effects is very difficult for researchers, as we all have a host of internal and external risk factors and exposures that can also lead to disease - but we should not ignore the current research in this new field that is beginning to link disease to shift work.

While this basic research will continue, the next phase will be - so what can we do to prevent disease linked to shift work? For now, all we can do is guess.

We know that patients will always need 24 hour care by nurses and other healthcare workers. So there will always be a night shift - and an evening shift. We know that nurses will always need and want to work, and will work off shifts. So for now, until research tells us better, we need to think how we can promote health for our off shift nurses. Not everyone who works off shift will get cancer - but we need to think about prevention for all, since we cannot separate the "wills" from the "will nots"!

We owe it to ourselves, both personally and as a profession, to keep up with the research on the health effects of shift work. We need to critically evaluate the literature and research findings, and adjust our systems and infrastructures to better support ourselves and our staff. This might potentially include offering nap times during the shift; adjusting the lighting; teaching staff about how to evaluate their personal risk factors and environmental risk factors in order to develop a life-plan that supports health.

For now, it has been suggested that shift workers try to maintain their shift routine 365 days per year - don't become a day person on days off and holidays. Sleep in the daytime without light - use blackout curtains and shades. Get a full amount of sleep daily, uninterrupted. Watch dietary intake to ensure it is healthy. Exercise. Try to get sources of UV light and vitamin D even when the sun is down. And these, really, are just guesses about what will make the night shift worker more likely to remain healthy and less likely to develop diseases like diabetes, CV disease and cancers. Until there is research to support interventions and preventive activities, use common sense, avoid fatigue, and monitor your health - including screening and that danged mammogram and Pap smear!

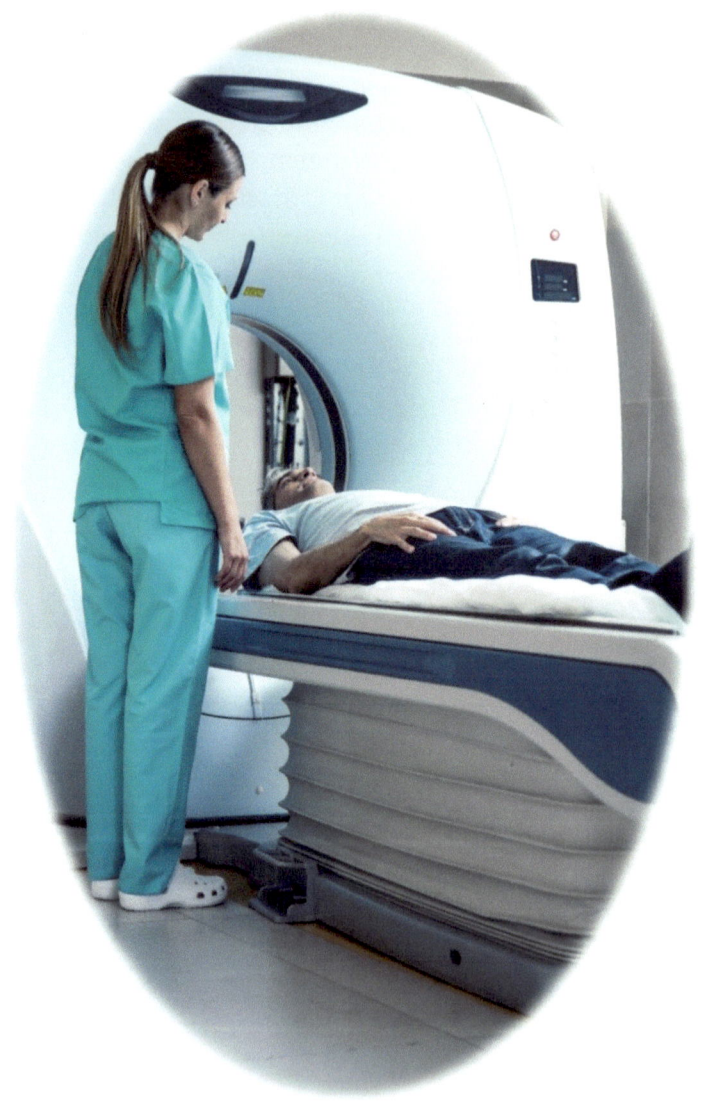

Informed consent for CT scans and X-rays?

My eyes were opened to the increased risk of cancer due to CT scans and other x-rays when I served on the Institutional Review Board (IRB) of a large University.

IRBs review research studies before they start, and at regular intervals thereafter, for the ethical and safe treatment of subjects and evidence of informed consent for study procedures and processes. I had never thought about any connection between radiology and cancer risk before my time on the IRB, even though I had sent hundreds of patients to radiology for x-rays and CT scans during my years as a clinical nurse, and had even had several x-rays and CT scans myself. As a patient, I was never told of any cancer risk associated with x-rays or CT scans, and as a nurse, I never taught patients about that risk - because I was unaware of it.

During my years on the IRB, I reviewed dozens of medical research studies for risks to subjects. And I became aware that for every single research study in which subjects had an exposure to ionizing radiation - from x-rays or CT scans - the investigators had to send paperwork to a special radiology committee that determined how much radiation each research subject would be exposed to for each particular radiological test in the study, and how that exposure increased their risk of developing cancer over their lifetime. This radiation exposure and increased risk of cancer were documented for each proposed study, and each research subject was told about this information. The potential subject could then ask questions, sign the consent to participate in the study, or refuse to participate, based on sound, unbiased information from radiology experts. This process was a true sign of informed consent, an important ethical principal in healthcare.

So I learned about the increased cancer risk through the IRB, but knew from my clinical experience that this same consideration was not given to patients in varied healthcare settings that I had worked at, in several different states in the U.S. Hmmmmm.

Now - I want you to ask yourself - was my experience as a clinical nurse unique, or does it happen every day in healthcare settings around the U.S.? I dare to say that it happens every single day - patients in healthcare settings and in the community are sent for radiological tests that expose them to ionizing radiation - without being informed that the test may increase their risk of developing cancer over their lifetime. I have heard tales of E.D.s where all trauma patients are routinely "CT'd" head to toe - no matter if there was trauma to their particular head (or toe!). And how about those community x-ray centers in local strip malls, where body scans are available for "only a few hundred bucks". Have you ever been tempted to walk in and get a body scan done? (I've been tempted!) How many patients with headaches or achy backs are exposed over and over again to ionizing radiation just because they complain of chronic pain, when past x-rays and scans have shown nothing significant or fixable? And how about children, whose bodies are still developing? What is their risk? And don't forget - patients with cancer are also routinely sent for regular follow-up CT scans to monitor the progress of tumors.

So....we know that we in healthcare routinely expose patients to ionizing radiation, that may increase their risk of developing cancer, WITHOUT INFORMED CONSENT. What does that mean?

According to this link, (http://health.usnews.com/health-news/patient-advice/articles/2015/03/06/imaging-tests-weighing-the-radiation-risk) 75 million CT scans are performed in the U.S. each year. The ionizing radiation dose in a CT scan is 500-600 times the amount in a chest x-ray. This study (http://health.usnews.com/health-news/blogs/second-opinion/2012/06/06/ct-scans-boost-cancer-risk-in-young-patients-study-finds) in Britain found that 2-3 CT head scans tripled a child's risk of getting a brain tumor. And that 5-10 scans that deliver radiation to the bone marrow increased the risk of developing leukemia. So, while radiation from CT scans and other x-rays might be considered small, children and adults who have repeated scans have been found to have a definite increased risk of cancer from the scans during their lifetime.

I am not writing to debate the science. I am sure that opinions and evidence abound on each side of this issue.

My question is this - shouldn't we use the same informed consent process that research studies are expected to use - with patients receiving healthcare services for medical, surgical and trauma conditions? That is, for every patient for whom a test is ordered that employs ionizing radiation (the type that increases cancer risk), providers should be mandated to offer an explanation of the amount of radiation that will be received, the implications of that radiation, and the amount of increased cancer risk over the patient's lifetime - and then the patient or decision-maker should sign an informed consent document for the ordered test.

We certainly must take into account that providers have the knowledge and ability to provide baseline numbers on the amount of radiation for each test in the Radiology Department, as well as the increased cancer risk related to that amount - but we also must teach patients that this risk is in addition to their baseline risk - which depends on their age, the background radiation that they are exposed to on a daily basis, and any excess radiation they have been exposed to due to altitude or employment, or even during airplane transportation. So it is not easy to be definitive that patient X will "get" cancer from his chest CT within the next 5 years - but can we not let patient X know that the ordered test does increase his cancer risk?

I myself have decided to skip the every-other-year head CT that I have been expected to have for my own medical condition. I have elected instead to choose an every year, less-invasive but still diagnostic and non-CT test instead, and to also pay close attention to any symptoms that I may be having. I truly believe that patients have the right to also make that decision for themselves, based on best-evidence information from their provider about the benefits and risks involved in the tests that are recommended for them. And that every provider has the ethical responsibility to provide that information to their patients as indicated for the tests that the provider orders. Order a risky test? Then inform the patient of the pros and cons and let them (or their decision maker) make an informed decision and give explicit consent. Don't be paternal and directive - be collaborative with your patients!

And for you non-prescribing nurses - consider having a discussion on this topic with your nursing department, with your Chief of Service, and with your ethics department. Decide what your own role will be in informing patients about the benefits and risks of tests - should you have a role? Should policy be changed at your facility? Explore the literature and the science, make your own informed decision about your nursing role, and follow through. Decide how you will act - I know that I already have.

- For more information, here is a link to a nice explanation of cancer risk from radiologic tests.

    - http://www.cancer.org/treatment/understandi ngyourdiagnosis/examsandtestdescriptions/i magingradiologytests/imaging-radiology-tests-rad-risk

- Also check out this site for adults

    - http://www.imagewisely.org/Patients

- [Here's an article](#) from the Mayo Clinic

  - http://www.ncbi.nlm.nih.gov/pmc/articles/PMC2996147/

- And one from [Penn Medicine](#).

  - http://www.oncolink.org/risk/article.cfm?c=12&id=17

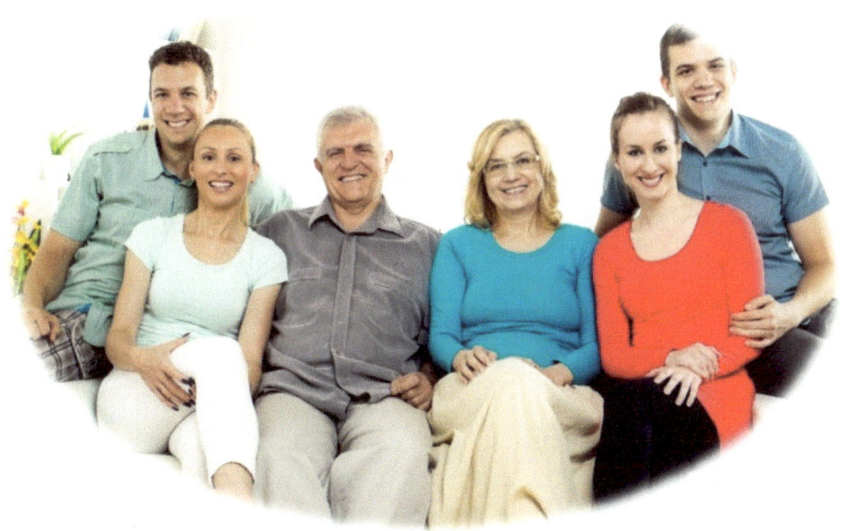

5 (well, 6) Fast Facts about STDs

STDs have been in the news quite frequently the past year or two. Gonorrhea. Chlamydia. Syphilis. HIV/AIDS. Herpes. HPV. Trichomoniasis. and others. Here are 5 fast facts that nurses should know about sexually transmitted diseases (also called sexually transmitted infections or STIs).

1. **STDs are becoming antibiotic resistant.** Strains of antibiotic resistant gonorrhea and syphilis are already seen in practice. As there is only one antibiotic class that gonorrhea is now susceptible to, prescribing habits for that infection have changed to try to prevent total resistance to that class of drug - the cephalosporins. Think about it - if this resistance continues to develop, gonorrhea, an STD that can lead to significant morbidity, may soon become a disease that has no cure. And how about syphilis, which when untreated affects the neurological system? Antibiotic resistance in STDs is concerning.

2. **Elders are sexually active and should be screened for STDs.** Even those in nursing homes. For my

dissertation research, I surveyed advanced practice nurses who provide women's health care. Several told me stories of sexual activity, and STDs, among the nursing home populations that they cared for. Moral of the story - have a high index of suspicion for STDs among the sexually active - even older adults. When the symptoms and behaviors fit, test for the disease! And screen, screen, screen! (and teach teach teach!)

PS - do not forget that HIV is also an STD - and elders can also be exposed to this infection through sexual activity or even from a blood transfusion in the early days of HIV - say early to mid-1980s before the blood supply was screened and cleaned for the disease. It has happened that older men who travel and who employ sex workers - and who, because of generational issues, have not been educated about STDs, HIV and transmission - unknowingly acquire the disease and then pass it on to their wife. Teaching the older at risk adult about STDs might be awkward, but is oh so very necessary!

3. **In the news this week - recommendations that screening for extra-vaginal STDs increase in at-risk women**. There are guidelines for men who have sex with men (MSM) for oral and rectal screening - but the recommendations have not been as strong for women. And yet women having sex with men and multiple partners have the same risks for extra-genital sexually transmitted diseases as MSM - oral and rectal infection. So if you care for sexually active women, teaching about STDs, risk prevention AND EXPECTED SCREENING (vaginal, oral and rectal) is vitally important. And if you are an APN, performing that screening is central to providing women's healthcare.

4. Remember, **HPV can cause cancer.** That is why the vaccine for that STD is so highly recommended for young people. But take your thoughts a step further - oral sex - infection - cancer. Rectal sex - infection - cancer. Actor Michael Douglas either did or did not acquire his throat cancer from oral sex - it's not clear to me if that was ever confirmed. But - it certainly could have happened. VACCINATE!

Trichomoniasis has been linked to prostate cancer- and chlamydia to DNA damage that leads to cancer. So STD education, prevention, screening and prompt treatment is important as a cancer preventative.

5. **About 20 million new STIs per year occur in the U.S.** Here are a few statistics from the CDC, 2013.

- 1,401,906 cases of chlamydia in 2013

- 333,004 cases of gonorrhea

- 17,275 cases of syphilis

- 348 cases of congenital syphilis

- While both males and females are at risk for STDs, females carry the higher risk of long-term consequences to health, including PID, pelvic pain, and infertility.

- The highest risk age group, who have 1/2 of the diagnosed cases, are between 15 and 24.

- MSM account for 3/4 of all primary and secondary syphilis cases, and about 1/2 of those cases are also infected with HIV.

6. **Do not forget education, prevention, screening and treatment for persons with a disability.**

Like older adults, persons with a disability may be perceived as asexual - but that is not a true perception. So for those of you dealing with the person with a new disability; with children born with a disability; AND for older adults with a newly acquired disability - remember to teach, screen and follow-up surveillance for STDs in those populations.

Nurses, no matter the setting, have a responsibility to screen for risk, and educate appropriate patients. And a responsibility to remain up to date on the latest in prevention and treatment for STDs.

For more information on recommended screenings, check out U.S. Preventive Services Task Force (USPSTF) Clinical Screening Guidelines at http://www.uspreventiveservicestaskforce.org/Page/Name/tools-and-resources-for-better-preventive-care

and the CDC at http://www.cdc.gov/std/prevention/screeningReccs.htm

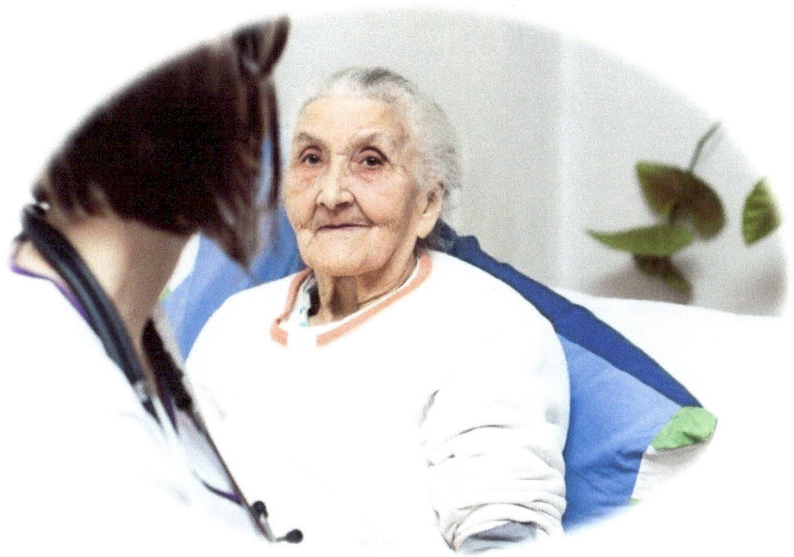

Restraints as fall prevention?

How does a nurse guarantee a family that their loved one won't fall? We know that falls are not preventable - and that nurses can't be everywhere at once. Probably one of my most memorable experiences as a nurse happened on my first job, on a 60 bed medical unit. Evening shift. Everyone but me, an aide, and a clerk had gone to the cafeteria. We heard a crash from the far end of the East hallway, and ran down to find a young girl having a seizure on the floor beside her bed. The roommate said that the girl had vaulted over the side rail during the seizure and landed on the floor. Luckily there were no injuries. And this was a totally unexpected, unavoidable fall.

Janice Morse PhD RN notes that there are three types of falls: unforeseeable, as above; predictable, as in the next paragraph; and preventable through attention to environment and other influences outside of the patient - such as water on the floor, clutter, and so on. So, if some are so predictable, let's prevent them with restraints - or not?

An aging family member has had multiple falls over several years. Currently 99 years old, she has poor balance; is prone to orthostatic hypotension; has poor vision; has sarcopenia (muscle wasting) with resultant decreased strength; and a propensity toward confusion.

The most recent falls resulted in a hairline ankle fracture managed with a splint; a black eye; and a femur fracture, hospitalization and ORIF. And last year? An ankle fracture and a cervical neck injury from sliding out of bed while trying to stand up. So for that she is also post-ankle ORIF and C-laminectomy. Right now, post hip-ORIF, she is confused, and an increased danger to herself as she tries to get up from bed. What is a family - and nurses - to do?

Of course, in the "olden days" (as our parents like to say), we freely used restraints as a fall prevention tool. Every nurse had that little Posey key on the blue plastic key fob in his or her pocket. And if we didn't use a locking belt, we used a vest with straps that tied into the bed frame - and, rarely, wrist restraints. I recall no cases of injury, added agitation, or problems with the use of restraints in that era. We gave good skin care, managed toileting assiduously, and made sure all restrained patients were fed, offered fluids, and gotten out of bed as much as possible. We gave excellent basic nursing care. And with that care, and with those restraints, our patients remained safe.

Now, of course, restraints are out of favor. It has been posited that restraints violate personal freedom, autonomy, and the ethical mandates of beneficence, nonmaleficence, and justice. Some have said that the application of restraints equals unlawful restraint, assault and battery. Restraints have been linked to significant morbidity, mortality and even PTSD. Physical injuries associated with restraint use include pressure ulcers, decrease in muscle mass and muscle tone (and thus strength and conditioning), urinary and fecal incontinence, orthostatic hypotension, bruising, increased risk of infection, DVT and PE, strangulation, contractures, and death from asphyxiation. Psychological effects may include fear, delirium, embarrassment, anxiety, depression, and damage to self-esteem.

First, restraints were replaced with sitters. But that was expensive. And research has shown that sitters do not necessarily prevent falls, and that the reduction of sitter use in facilities does not change fall rates. Now, multiple other interventions are being attempted in healthcare facilities in order to prevent falls and maintain safety. One thing facilities cannot afford is to increase the number of staff. Funding agencies do not like to pay for extra help, either. And if a staff member is pulled from one assigned area to care for a single patient, without that staff member being replaced, patients in the now under-staffed area are at higher risk of injury. There are no easy answers.

So, yes, there are legal, ethical and practical - and facility and cost and personnel - issues all tied up with fall prevention. YIKES!

We know that nurses and other providers have a responsibility for fall prevention AND to those who may be considered for restraint use. When a patient is identified as high fall risk due to agitation and/or confusion, the first responsibility is safety - the second is to determine the cause of agitation and delirium. For more on this, please see the module on delirium at www.nurs-ed.com/confusion

Here are a few suggestions:

Before any type of restraint, chemical or physical, is given or applied for fall prevention, have you:

1. assessed the cause of the agitation and/or confusion? Is it medical? Is it pain? Is it a need for toileting? Human contact? Food and fluids? Skin care? Is there a need for a medication review?

2. tried changing the environment? Worked on sleep patterns? Provided a minimally confusing environment by reducing the noise and chaos in the patient area? Added calendars and clocks to the room? Natural light? Minimized tethers, tubes and lines?

3. Have you lowered the bed? Provided padded side rails? Tried a lap belt with a hook and loop release?

4. Have you tried distraction by way of an activity backpack, simple puzzles, folding laundry, sorting papers, walking, going outside?

5. Tried adding cameras with remote visualization, increasing frequency of rounding, or recliner chairs?

5. Checked out the following resources?

o ANA Position Statement on Restraint and Seclusion in Health Care Settings

   o http://www.nursingworld.org/restraintposition

- o Multiple resources from the Hartford Institute for Geriatric Nursing

    - o http://consultgerirn.org/searched?q=restraints& Submit_search.x=0&Submit_search.y=0

- o Use of physical restraints in neurosurgery: a guide for good practice

    - o http://www.intechopen.com/books/explicative-cases-of-controversial-issues-in-neurosurgery/use-of-physical-restraints-in-neurosurgery-guide-for-a-good-practice

- o Reducing restraint use for adults in acute care

    - o http://journals.lww.com/nursing/Fulltext/2013/12000/Reducing_restraint_use_for_older_adults_in_acute.18.aspx#P11

I am not sure what we will do with our own family member. I do think that, if restraints are employed as a safety measure for any patient, that basic, competent, caring nursing care is the key to preventing morbidity and mortality related to restraints. We cannot "tie people up" and then never check on them again! Sometimes basic nursing care is denigrated and pushed aside as too simple - and even trusted to untrained personnel and untrained families - but, you know, it is undoubtedly the most important aspect of nursing and is certainly the basis for all of healthcare and healing.

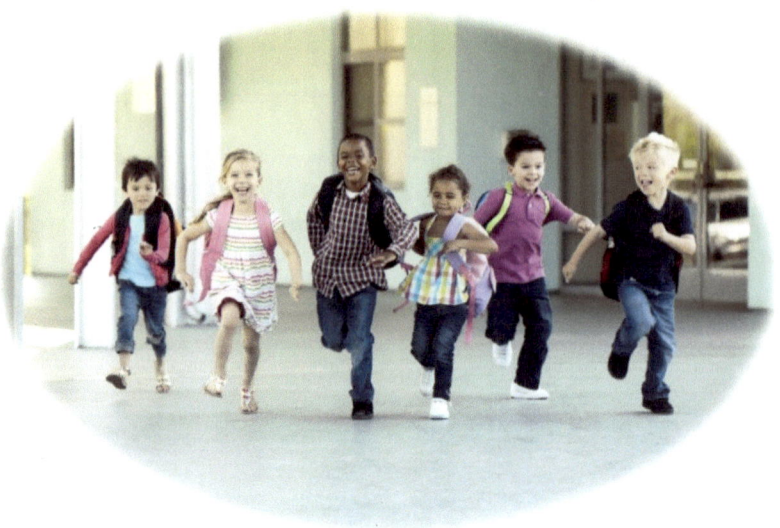

The human microbiome

If you have been paying attention to the news lately, you have been hearing more and more about the human microbiome, specifically the bacteria in our gut. There has been a wealth of research on this topic making its way into the popular lay-literature - aka our local newspapers and magazines. It's fascinating!

Researchers are looking to find the connection between the human microbiome and health and disease. The federal government opened the Human Microbiome Project in 2008. Here's a link to this fascinating work (http://commonfund.nih.gov/hmp/index). There are some great resources on that website, and articles and podcasts about findings such as **"Researchers Show Premature Infants Can Develop Sepsis From Gut Microbes"** and more.

Seems like there are somewhere in the neighborhood of 100 trillion bacteria and other microbes - something like a thousand strains of bacteria - in and on the human body that play a role in organ function, health and disease. These bacteria are essential for digestion, repelling noxious invaders, and other yet unknown activities. And each person's personal microbiome is different from every other person's. These original microbiomes may explain why people react differently to medications, or why some people are more susceptible to certain types of infection. Asthma, obesity, bowel and other diseases may someday be explained by "microbiomes gone awry".

Some have suggested that humans are the packaging, the suitcase, for the vast number of microbes we carry. Yucky thought! It's long been known that babies born by C-section are more likely to exhibit some problem with immunity that make them more prone to celiac disease, allergies, eczema, asthma and maybe even Type 1 diabetes - it's now thought that the microbes picked up from Mom during a vaginal delivery are essential in establishing the right microbe mix on the skin, in the gut and elsewhere are needed for normal immune function throughout life. Babies born vaginally develop a biome that resembles the biome of the mother's vagina - those born by C-section develop a biome that resembles the mother's skin. During pregnancy, the biome of the mother's vagina changes to include more *Lactobacillus,* necessary for digestion of milk. A baby born by C-section does not receive inoculation with *Lactobacillus* and thus may have more difficulty with the digestion of milk from Mom. It may be that transmission of mother's vaginal bacteria onto newborns during birth acts as a defense against future disease by limiting the colonization of more harmful pathogens. And, note this - this effect of the composition of the gut bacteria has been found to last at least 7 years.

One other associated topic that has hit the news recently is fecal transplants. That brought you an immediate visual, didn't it! The goal of fecal transplants is to take a sample of a healthy gut microbiome from someone who meets certain criteria, and transfer that sample of microbes to someone with a specific disease - such as c diff. A word of caution - search fecal transplant on Google and you will come up with self-help sites that instruct people how to do this at home. Oh, my. Not recommended for a number of reasons! But, back to c-diff - the thought is that antibiotic use in vulnerable patients causes depletion of beneficial microbes - which leads to proliferation of clostridium difficile - but a fecal transplant with a healthy microbiome will replace these microbes and result in a cure ~90% of the time (http://www.mayoclinic.org/medical-professionals/clinical-updates/digestive-diseases/quick-inexpensive-90-percent-cure-rate).

Much is yet to be seen as to the effects of the gut microbes on disease - but I think that before I would accept a fecal transplant I would have to know how it is prepared! I have heard that in some studies the microbes have been put into capsules that are swallowed - but the Mayo site talks about colonoscopies and ng tubes being used to introduce the transplant. Hmmmmmm.

Have you watched the related TV ads recently? When yogurt companies and health food corporations tell us about the microbes they add to their products to help our health and digestion? If you stop and think about it, it might be a bit troubling - if we have a thousand or more strains of microbes here, there and everywhere on our body, can taking a single supplement with one or two or three of these make a difference? Who know which microbes any particular person is missing? Who knows what mix of microbes is best for health? Who knows what dosage or strength of microbe is needed to treat a condition? Who knows the difference in microbiomes and needs depending on age, gender, race or genetic make-up? The answers, of course, are not yet known.

Whatever the case, I believe that the field of research concerning the human microbiome will affect nursing practice in years to come, as more links to disease are discovered. Keep your eye to the professional and lay literature for updates on research findings!

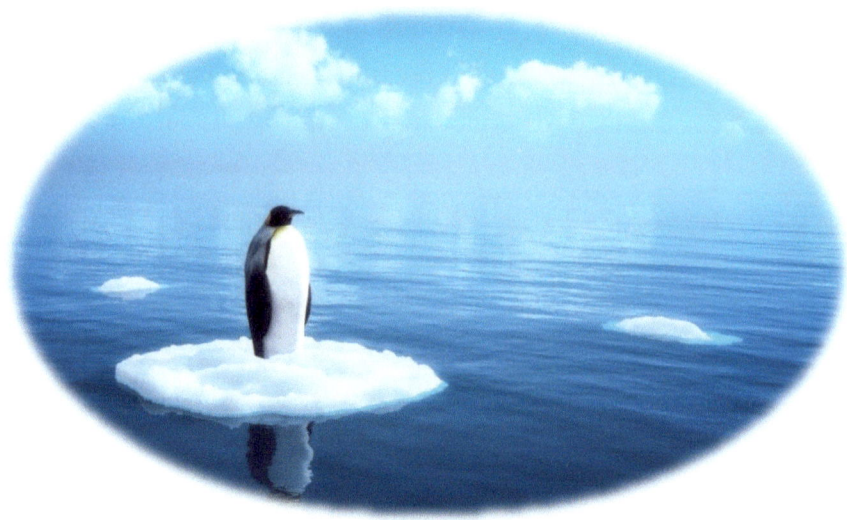

Climate change

Climate change is upon us. Sometimes, I feel like the only one in my vicinity who is terrified of its effects.

We see in the news, on the internet, and in our social media that there are many people who deny its presence. There are nurses in my Facebook friends list who loudly share their non-belief left and right. But, you know, it is not a case of denial.

You might as well deny that the sun comes up in the morning or that the sky is blue. Climate change IS. It's a FACT. It's science. It's here, it's now, and the effects are worsening by the day. So what, you say? What does that have to do with nursing and healthcare? Great question!

"In 2008, the International Council of Nurses position statement (2008) on Nurses, Climate Change and Health argues that "climate change is an important issue for the nursing profession, particularly in light of the impact on people's health and nursing's shared responsibility to sustain and protect the natural environment from depletion, pollution, degradation and destruction". It called on nurses to help prevent the impact of climate change on those groups most vulnerable to injury, including the elderly, the

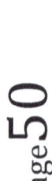

poor, and socially isolated city dwellers."
(http://www.academia.edu/1517598/Climate_change_and_
nursing_why_nursing_may_duck_the_issue)

The American Nurses Association recognizes climate change as a human and environmental threat. You can find more information at http://www.nursingworld.org/MainMenuCategories/Workp laceSafety/Healthy-Work-Environment/Environmental-Health/Issues/Climate

The issues

Average Weather Conditions: According to the EPA: "Changes in climate affect the average weather conditions that we are accustomed to. Warmer average temperatures will likely lead to hotter days and more frequent and longer heat waves. This could increase the number of heat-related illnesses and deaths. Increases in the frequency or severity of extreme weather events such as storms could increase the risk of dangerous flooding, high winds, and other direct threats to people and property. Warmer temperatures could increase the concentrations of unhealthy air and water pollutants. Changes in temperature, precipitation patterns, and extreme events could enhance the spread of some diseases."

Coping with Weather: I don't know about you, but I live in Texas. I have evacuated my home for storms – and even moved away from the coast because my husband "had a feeling" that Galveston was due for a hurricane – and it hit a year after we left. Those weather events, alone – severe weather and population evacuation – are the source for new research into the effects on people. Older adults in particular suffer from changes in environment – and think about New Orleans and Katrina – I suggest that you read "5 Days at Memorial" by Sheri Fink to get a feel for what it is like to be in the aftermath of a severe weather event. And for those who evacuate? Well, think about the logistics – where do you get your medicine? Your oxygen? Your food? Your dialysis – in a strange place, with no healthcare provider that knows you? What about the stress of being stranded on the highway – your dog dead in the back seat from the heat, your kids dehydrated, dizzy and somnolent? Who pays for the gas when you didn't have money in the first place? And, how do you find a shelter if you don't know the area?

Morbidity and mortality increase in severe weather events, from exposure to the weather; from evacuation; from exacerbation of pre-existing disease; from stress; from social issues; from psychological issues; from hygiene issues; from crime.

Climate change affects air quality – increases in ozone, fine particulates, smog. Think about your patients with pre-existing pulmonary problems like asthma, emphysema and chronic bronchitis. Where do they go to find fresh air? Can they afford multiple trips to the specialist, or repeated hospitalizations? How about children who play outside – the exposures are not good for their lung health. Go on the web and learn about pollution in China and then imagine that in your part of the world.

Climate change will affect food borne diseases as well – Here's more from the EPA "Higher air temperatures can increase cases of salmonella and other bacteria-related food poisoning because bacteria grow more rapidly in warm environments. These diseases can cause gastrointestinal distress and, in severe cases, death. [1]

Flooding and heavy rainfall can cause overflows from sewage treatment plants into fresh water sources. Overflows could contaminate certain food crops with pathogen-containing feces"

Yuk. It was just this week that the news went crazy over feces and toilet paper being found in the cilantro supply. Think about the recent massive rain and floods in the South and elsewhere. This mess is closer than we admit!

Water-borne Parasites: Like to go to the lake? Think again! "Heavy rainfall or flooding can increase water-borne parasites such as *Cryptosporidium* and *Giardia* that are sometimes found in drinking water. These parasites can cause gastrointestinal distress and in severe cases, death.

Heavy rainfall events cause storm water runoff that may contaminate water bodies used for recreation (such as lakes and beaches) with other bacteria. The most common illness contracted from contamination at beaches is gastroenteritis, an inflammation of the stomach and the intestines that can cause symptoms such as vomiting, headaches, and fever. Other minor illnesses include ear, eye, nose, and throat infections."

Population effects of climate change: Climate change is already causing droughts, floods, melting ice caps, impacts on wildlife and coastal cities, excessive temperature fluctuations.....Buffalo, NY still has piles of snow around the city (it is August as I write this!!). Population impacts will soon be seen – and are expected to include problems with our agriculture and food supply; migration and immigration; disease and death; aggression and war; jobs (no farms, no employment, etc).

And there are many more issues, too many to review here. But all are pretty scary.

So what can we do as nurses?

- Accept that climate change exists. Believe the science.

- Pay attention to the news. Make it your goal to learn more about the topic.

- Adopt a low carbon lifestyle

- Learn more about your personal food supply and its safety

- Pay attention to weather patterns in your area

- Have an evacuation plan

- Look around your community – who and what are at risk?

  o Think about volunteering in community efforts like supplying fans in the summer, blankets and coats in the winter, barriers to flood waters, etc.

- Get involved with your community's emergency planners. Advocate for the elderly, poor, and otherwise vulnerable in your community.

- Work with local health officials in preparedness activities.

- Get the "climate change" issue into nursing education – at the university curricular level, in nursing organizations, and in your local healthcare facilities. Demand education and action about climate change where you work.

- Get involved in policy – talk to your local, state and national legislators on the topic. Advocate through government for responsible policy regarding climate change.

Nurses should accept climate change as a fact, treat it as a personal threat to themselves as a world citizen, and find out how they can be engaged in addressing the issue. Not to sound overly morbid, but there will come a time when it is too late to act.

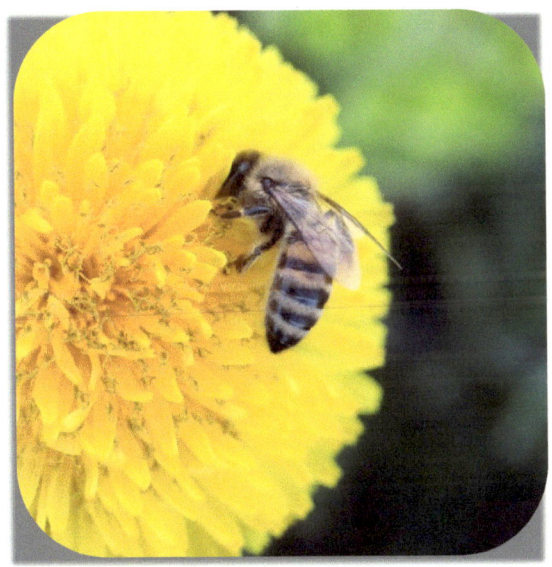

www.ingramcontent.com/pod-product-compliance
Lightning Source LLC
Chambersburg PA
CBHW040900180526
45159CB00001B/474